Immune System Diet & Lifestyle
The Best Foods, Drinks, Natural Remedies & Holistic Recipes to Stay Healthy & Prevent Disease

(Immune System Boosters Book 1)

By Elena Garcia

Copyright ©Elena Garcia 2020

www.YourWellnessBooks.com

All cooking is an experiment in a sense, and many people come to the same or similar recipe over time. All recipes in this book have been derived from author's personal experience. Should any bear a close resemblance to those used elsewhere, that is purely coincidental.

any health or medical issues – you should be talking to your doctor first.

Contents

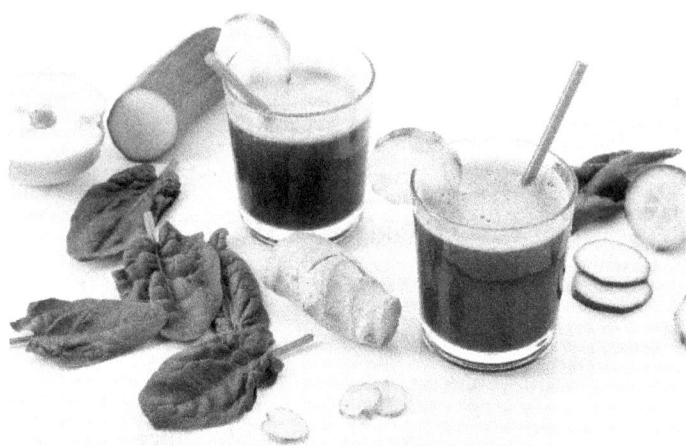

Introduction: From Fear to Freedom

We all want to stay healthy, vibrant, and energized. And we all want to feel confident knowing we are doing the right things to give our body what it needs to thrive.

The problem? Life can get busy and stressful. And when it does, we tend to put our health and self-care at the end of our "to-do-lists." Sometimes, we don't pay any attention to our health until we get a wake-up call (usually manifesting as a disease).

The good news? Taking care of your body through healthy habits and balanced lifestyle choices doesn't have to be hard. There are many effective diet tweaks that are simple to implement and have the power to strengthen your immune system.

So that you get sick less, and even when you do, you recover faster! As your body gets stronger and you start noticing the effects of your healthy choices, you develop more confidence in your body and its ability to heal.

The main reason why I decided to write this book is to empower you. Yes, I know you are busy! And I know that being 100% perfect with your diet, or following the latest "health fad" is not only impossible but also impractical.

Luckily, with the help of this little book, you can start taking meaningful action step-by-step. Each tip outlined in this book will tell you what you need to focus on (whether it's a superfood or a herb) and how to use it in real life (we are talking an abundance of recipes you can pick and choose from).

I love empowering my readers, and I love giving them different choices as well! So, this guide is not that much about following a specific diet. Instead, it's more about tweaking your current diet and lifestyle by making a few simple shifts to benefit your immune system.

So that you feel energized and get sick less. And so that you feel confident knowing you can take care of your body while doing everything you possibly can to keep it healthy.

Please note- the keyword here is "everything you POSSIBLY CAN." We are not talking about some magical cure books. Also, this book is not aimed at diagnosing or treating any health issues. It's not a medical book, and I am not your physician. As a wellness writer, I know my place, and ethical framework is critical to me. I don't like the hype, overnight miracles, or marketing claims.

This book focuses on empowerment, healthy lifestyle choices, and prevention through giving your body natural foods that are rich in substances that have been scientifically proven to strengthen your immune system.

And this my friend is true empowerment. You are focusing on what you can do instead of living in fear, neglect, or negativity.

Being positive is not only about positive thinking. It's more about taking positive action- whenever you can, to the best of your ability!

This book is your wellness self-help guide. You can start helping your body right here and right now. And you can do the best you can to make it stronger!

At the same time, please remember to visit your doctor regularly for checkups and blood work, etc. (even if you are healthy). That way, any imbalances or deficiencies can get detected earlier rather than later, and the path to recovery and healing can be much shorter. If you suffer from any existing health issues or are on medication, I highly recommend you consult your diet and lifestyle choices with your doctor.

"Oh, but come on, if it's natural, it's always good for me and safe, right?". Yes, most of the time, it is, especially if you are healthy and don't have any allergies and are not on medication.

But, you always want to make sure you stay on the safe side. Some natural herbs may interfere with certain medications, and some superfoods (even if they work great for 99.9999% of people who use them) may just not the right choice for you and your body.

11

Introduction

The best thing you can do for yourself is to combine the natural world and self-education (like, for example, this book or other wellness self-help guides like this one) with science and expertise from your health care provider or medical professional.

With that being said (or written, lol!), let's have a look what is covered in this little booklet!

The Immune System Diet & Lifestyle book is a simple blueprint you can follow even on a busy schedule, without having to buy expensive supplements or gadgets.

One tool I recommend you get though is a blender to make smoothies and soups. Juicer is optional. For all the juicing recipes included in this book, even a simple lemon squeezer will do, so you don't need to worry about buying a juicer (unless you want to, or already have one).

This guide is designed to help you improve your diet and lifestyle in a few simple steps you can quickly implement in a week (or less).

Here's What You Will Find Inside the Immune System Diet & Lifestyle book:

- The absolute immune system basics nobody talks about and the most affordable way to turn your body into a health-generating machine.

- Why it's not only about what you eat and the best drinks to feed your body with vital micronutrients to fight disease, stay healthy and feel energized.
- THE SIMPLEST diet tweak to help your body heal and stay in balance (and why MOST diets overlook it).
- How to rest, even if your work schedule or family obligations don't allow you to be a sleepyhead (plus the best natural remedies and tips to relax let go and maximize your rest routine, without having to sleep more).
- The MOST immune system boosting foods you can easily find in your local supermarket inexpensively (and how to add them to your diet in a few simple steps) plus - RECIPES INCLUDED
- Foods to AVOID or REDUCE as well as the most pro-inflammatory, immune-suppressing, hormone-unbalancing food you are probably consuming every day (without even realizing it's destroying your body's natural ability to heal).
- Why the "Wash your hands, use sanitizer, don't shake hands, don't hug, don't go to big public gatherings, reconsider travel plans..." (even though great) may not be enough unless you do this one thing (and focus on the internal change).
- THE MOST EFFECTIVE immune-system boosting, all-natural recipes (MOST of which you can make in 10-15 minutes or less).

- BONUS – MY #1 HEALTH SECRET I discovered by accident + how it saves me $1000 a year (or MORE) while making me losing weight almost effortlessly and improving my (and my family's) wellbeing.

Plus much, much MORE to help you live a healthy, safe, and empowered lifestyle while giving your body what it needs to stay disease-free and strong!

The 3 Pillars of Vibrant Health

It all starts with empowerment. That inner feeling that maybe there is something you can do to help yourself. That perhaps, there is something more out there. That maybe, you can transform your body and mind and become a healthier version of yourself.

And congrats to You, My Friend! If you are reading this book, chances are you are already empowered!

For some reason, you decided to let go of skepticism, and you picked up this little booklet because you believe in yourself, and you know you can help yourself.

Most people never take this step. They believe that things just happen. They think there is good luck and bad luck, or that it's all about genetics. And, yes, there is some truth to that. As I already said, we can't control everything. But-true empowerment is all about focusing on what we can do, right here and right now.

I don't know about You, but I leave the rest to the Higher Power and prayer (I don't want to get too philosophical here, so I will just skip this part for now). The bottom line is – always focus on what you can control and see adverse circumstances as a challenge to make you stronger and motivate you to do something different.

This is what I like to call the True Empowerment!

And this is our First Pillar of Health. When you feel empowered, you focus on what you can control. And what you focus on expands.

You see, your mind works like a search engine. Imagine you go on Google and YouTube and type in a diet, let's say it's the keto diet or some other diet. You can type in "keto success stories," to see how it worked for other people and how much weight they have lost. Or you can type in "keto scam," or something else. Both are fine. There is no right or wrong.

The only thing I want you to pay attention to is your mind and how it works. If you focus on why something will not work for you and is not worth doing -your mind (just like a Google search engine), will find the evidence to back it up.

And at the same time, if you focus on why something does work, you will also find the evidence to back it up as well.

What you decide to focus on is up to you! Personally, I always intend to focus on the positive, while not staying ignorant of the negative. For example, while studying a new herb, I want to be open to all its amazing health benefits, but I also want to know the possible side effects to stay on the safe side.

However, I don't choose to focus on the negative 100%, because that would make me depressed, and I would never do or try anything new to improve my health.

Unfortunately, some people are like that. Nothing can spark their interest. Exercise is not worth it; healthy herbal teas are not worth it; eating more vegetables and fruits is not worth it.

Yes, we will all die. But, as long as we are here, why not enjoy energy and vitality and be grateful for the fact that we are here? Why not show the God, the Universe/ the Higher Power (whatever your belief is) that because we are grateful we are here- we do the best we can, whenever we can so that we can take care of ourselves?

Stay empowered and inspired by focusing on what you can control, right here, right now!

The second pillar of health is..

Taking Inspired Action backed up by patience and belief.

No action, no results. It's as simple as that! Now, I will be the first one to admit that I have been guilty of paralysis by analysis. I like reading and researching. And so, I spent many years just reading about weight loss and different diets, but would never take action on the information I studied! Until one day, I had a wake-up call. I was on a weight loss forum, and I got involved in a discussion about a diet X and why it works and why diet Y was better. I was there, kind of trolling around and sharing my opinions in a negative way.

Until this young fit girl, who was a weight loss coach, asked me- *Ok, if you know so much about it, please tell us how much weight you lost and how many people you helped to lose weight. Otherwise, stop talking about the things you haven't done yourself. You are just judging and criticizing others!*

At first, I felt so pissed off. How come, this young girl, who probably doesn't have all this knowledge that I have is telling me what to do?

Well, she was right, and she put me in my place. I was just talking about the things I have read about in books, but I have never tried any of them.

Now, I am a different person, and I don't get involved in internet discussions about nutrition. And, even if I did, I would only share my own experience based on what I did and what worked or didn't work (and I would be kind to others).

So, from my own experience, and mindset transformation, I can honestly tell you that taking action (even imperfect) is all you need to focus on. When you read about this great superfood, ask yourself: *Ok, so how can I add it to my diet, quickly and painlessly?*

It doesn't have to be all or nothing. But, unfortunately, in our health community, many people go for all or nothing. I am super healthy and eat 100% clean (or follow this new diet 100%), or I eat fast food and tell myself that staying healthy is too hard!

The choice is always yours; you can always choose. But my number one tip for you is – take imperfect massive action and just do something today. Show your mind that you work with it, not against it. Nobody is perfect; it's not about being perfect; it's about PROGRESS!

So, to sum up, our first pillar is Empowerment. Then, we have to take Meaningful Action (the best we can, while letting go of perfection).

Finally, the Third Pillar is KISS!

Keep It Super Simple!

We are talking simple recipes and habits that will make your healthy lifestyle super enjoyable and fun! The KISS methods in this book are specifically designed to help you strengthen your immune system and enjoy a healthy, stress-free, and energized life.

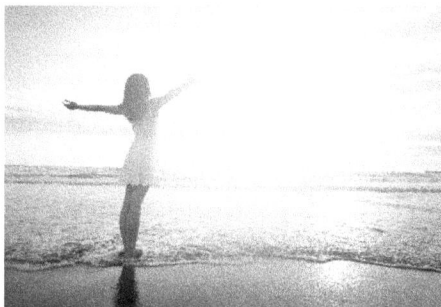

First Things First – Why Your Immune System Should Be Your Number One Focus

When it comes to protecting yourself from diseases and viruses, you already know the following:

Wash your hands, use sanitizer, avoid shaking hands and hugging...etc

Great advice for sure...But- you already know this!

The problem is that nobody is talking about the most important thing you can do, which is to strengthen and fortify your immune system.

Why?

Why Your Immune System Is Important And What It Does

The role of the immune system is to protect your body from any foreign matters or substances that might cause any damage or imbalance while damaging the homeostasis. The effectiveness of your immune system depends on its ability to discriminate between foreign (nonself) and host(self) cells. When an organism is threatened by viruses or other harmful microorganisms, the immune system acts to provide protection.

Usually, the immune system does not initiate a response against self.

At the same time, the lack of an immune response is called tolerance.

When a foreign matter or a virus enters your body, your defense system recognizes this as foreign through the immune system. Each cell in your body carries a mixture of proteins and sugars that serve to identify the cell to the immune system. Foreign objects lack the identifiers that all of the body's cells have, but each one has unique features or antigens where the immune system attaches identifiers called antibodies.

This is the basis for the specific defense mechanisms.

Once you have built the antibodies for a specific antigen, the immune system will respond faster than if there had been no previous exposure to the antigen (i.e. you are immune to the pathogen, but only that specific pathogen, because your immune system responds faster.)

The non-specific part of the immune system is mostly composed of phagocytes (eating-cells), which engulf and digest foreign substances like bacteria and viruses, which do not bear the body's specific identifiers.

There is SO Much You Can Do to Protect Yourself from Viruses by Strengthening Your Immune System

It's time for you to discover the absolute immune system superfoods basics you have to start today (even if you are busy), including:

-The most immune-boosting foods to add in

-The most immune-suppressing foods to eliminate or reduce

-My BEST immune-boosting recipes to start using today (such as delicious and cleverly designed smoothies!)

So, let's get started and get your body strong, healthy, and protected as much as possible!

Your beautiful immune system is so powerful and effective (when given the right fuel and taken care of).

It is so smart! It is vital to so many functions in your body, and most importantly – what you eat, drink, and your lifestyle directly impacts how well it functions and how well it protects you from foreign invaders that can result in disease.

Here's the sad truth...When you are stressed, and you have been eating a processed fast-food diet while getting poor sleep, you're more likely to pick up a bug, cough, cold or the flu.

And when you get sick and your body is unhealthy, it takes much longer to heal and recover.

Also, when it comes to viruses...If they attack your body, your immune system will try to defend it.

If your immune system is compromised, then you stand more chance of succumbing to illness. If it's healthy, it will have a better chance of fighting it off. Simple, right?

So, let's start now with the Immune System Quartet!

(aka the absolute basics to help you boost your immune system)

These are especially important in winter or during every flu season.

The Immune System Quartet

Here's what your body needs to stay strong:

-Vitamin C,

-Zinc,

-Curcumin,

-Vitamin D

And yes, you could just take some supplements and be done with the rest of this book.

But, here's one thing to understand: quality supplements from reputable brands can be costly. At the same time, even the most expensive and quality supplements can't guarantee proper absorption. If your body is out of balance, chances are, some vitamins and supplements may not absorb properly. Or, you may overdo them and imbalance something else.

Don't get me wrong- I have nothing against supplements and vitamins. But, I would turn to them only if recommended and prescribed by my doctor (as the last remedy).

The good news is that you can feed your body with an abundance of Vitamin C, as well as zinc, curcumin, and

Vitamin D, by optimizing your nutrition. If that step doesn't help, and if your blood work will prove you are deficient in any of the vitamins mentioned above and nutrients, then talk to your doctor about supplementation.

If you are already taking any supplements and having success with it- keep it up.

All I want to open your eyes to is the power of natural and balanced nutrition. These are the immune system basics that can be implemented quite affordably (and naturally).

Multiple studies have proven all four of these to be effective in preventing, reducing the severity and reducing the length of colds & flu, because they directly support the immune system.

VITAMIN C

Since bodies do not produce or store the water-soluble vitamin C., we need to replenish our supply of vitamin C every day. The best natural source is from fruits and vegetables, especially the following:

-orange,

-kiwi,

-lemon,

-guava,

- grapefruit,

-broccoli,

-cauliflower,

-Brussel sprouts

-red bell peppers

-papaya

-strawberries

-cantaloupe

I recommend going for fresh, seasonal fruits and veggies. Also, when it comes to fruit, my personal choice is to focus on low sugar fruits (such as lemons or grapefruits) more than other fruit that is rich in sugar (such as oranges or kiwis).

Of course, it's all about balance. But, I like to make sure I follow a low sugar diet for the most part.

So, now that you are being reminded about the importance of Vitamin C, have a look at your diet and lifestyle and ask yourself – *Am I eating enough fruits and veggies?*

I'll be the first one to admit and be 100% honest with you. I am not the best fruit and veggie eater. Yes, you heard me right, I don't actually eat that many fruits of veggies.

Yea, I know, it kind of makes me fake for writing this book. I am exposing myself. I told you I don't take any vitamins and that natural foods is where it's at. And now, I am telling you I am not the most disciplined fruit and veggie eater!

But...I still get plenty of them in my diet! You see, I am a REAL SMOOTHIE monster! So, smoothie is my number one tool to make sure I get enough of fruits and veggies.

I usually drink a massive, Vitamin-C rich smoothie in the morning. Below, you will find my favorite Vitamin-C rich smoothies of all kinds. Some of them are fruit smoothies, some sneak in some greens (also great for you, more on that later), some veggies, and natural protein to help me stay full for hours.

Set a simple goal – start your day with a massive, vitamin-rich smoothie. Just get it done first thing in the morning. Store any left-overs for later, if needed. Also, whenever you feel like snacking some unhealthy, or processed, have a big smoothie instead!

Ever since I focused on smoothies (normally 1 smoothie a day), my sugar cravings almost evaporated!. Also, as I mentioned before, I am very mindful about high-sugar fruit, and so, I focus mostly on low sugar, Vitamin C rich foods. Real game changer!

Vitamin C Rich Smoothie Recipes

Vitamin C Happy Mind Smoothie

This smoothie combines spinach and grapefruits to help you enjoy more energy. Grapefruit, just like limes and lemons, is very low in sugar and high alkaline minerals such as Magnesium (to make your immune system even stronger!).

Serves: 1-2
Ingredients
Liquid:
- 2 cups coconut water, unsweetened

Dry:
- 1 small avocado, peeled, pitted and sliced
- Half cup mixed greens washed
- 1 big grapefruit, peeled and cut into smaller pieces
- 2 tablespoons sunflower seeds

Instructions
1. Place all the ingredients in a blender.
2. Process well until smooth. Enjoy!

Quinoa Alkaline Protein Smoothie

Quinoa makes this smoothie super-filling and adds some natural protein. You can even use this recipe as a quick brunch, lunch or a healthy, Vitamin C rich meal replacement for detox and health.

Serves: 1-2
Ingredients
Liquid:
- 1 cup coconut milk, unsweetened
- Juice of 1 lemon

Dry:
- 5 big tablespoons of quinoa, cooked and cooled down
- 1 big cucumber, peeled and cut into smaller pieces
- 1 small garlic clove, peeled

Other:
- A big handful of cilantro leaves washed
- A pinch of Himalayan salt
- A pinch of cumin powder
- A pinch of curry powder

Instructions
1. Blend all the ingredients in a blender. Serve and enjoy!

When Life Throws Lemons Smoothie

This smoothie is just perfect on a hot summer day. It will help you stay refreshed and energized.

Serves: 2-3
Ingredients
Liquid:
- 1 cup almond milk
- 1 cup of coconut water

Dry:
- 2 small limes, peeled and cut into smaller pieces
- 2 tablespoons chia seeds

Other:
- 1 teaspoon cinnamon powder
- 1 cup of ice cubes
- Stevia to sweeten, if needed

Instructions:
1. Place everything in a blender.
2. Process until smooth. Serve and enjoy!
3. Serve chilled and enjoy! This smoothie also makes a great morning detox drink.

Vitamin C Sweetness Smoothie

This recipe creates the perfect balance by combining citric fruit with natural sweetness that dates and watermelon offer. I love this smoothie on a hot summer day.

Servings: 2

Ingredients:

- 1 big grapefruit, peeled and chopped
- 1 lime, peeled
- A few dates, pitted
- 1 cup fresh watermelon chunks
- 1 cup of coconut water
- A few mint leaves to garnish

Instructions:

1. Place all the ingredients in a blender.
2. Process until smooth.
3. Serve in a smoothie glass and garnish with a few mint leaves.
4. Drink to your health and enjoy!

Super Veggie Smoothie

The combination of spinach and sweet peppers in this smoothie is another example of how the body's ability to absorb the high iron content of the spinach is boosted by pairing it with another vegetable that is high in vitamin C. This smoothie can also be enjoyed as a nice, raw, or warm healing soup.

Servings: 2
Ingredients:

- 1 cup fresh baby spinach leaves
- 1 red bell pepper, sliced
- A handful of raw pistachios, roughly chopped
- Half of a ripe avocado
- 1 cup coconut or nut milk of your choice
- Half cup of water, filtered, preferably alkaline
- Himalaya salt to taste (optional)

Instructions:

1. Place all the ingredients in a blender.
2. Process until smooth.
3. If needed, add more water.
4. Enjoy!

To give you more Vitamin C-rich smoothie ideas:

-red bell peppers blend great with coconut milk, or nut milk, cinnamon and a few slices of avocado and lime

-kiwis blend well with all kinds of greens as well as blueberries and garlic

-oranges taste amazing with avocados and nut milk (especially if you like creamy smoothies!)

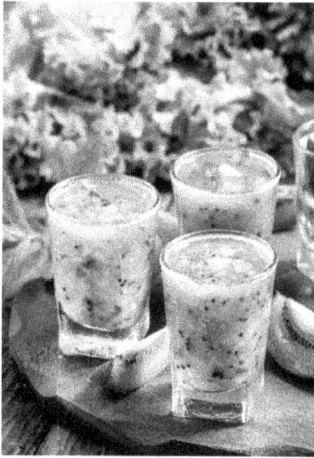

Now, back to the rest of the ingredients from our Immune System Quartet...

Zinc

Zinc metabolizes nutrients while maintaining your immune system and growing/ repairing your body tissues.

Your body doesn't store zinc, so you need to eat enough every day to ensure you're meeting your daily requirements.

There are many delicious zinc-rich foods you can add to your diet (both plant-based and animal-based), such as:

1. Meat and shellfish.
2. Legumes (great alternative for vegans and vegetarians).
3. Seeds and nuts.
4. Eggs.
5. Dark chocolate and cocoa (yummy!)

So now, let's have a look at some quick, zinc-rich recipes (including some yummy salads!).

Also, please note, if you really took to smoothies (and I hope you did), you can start adding some zinc-rich foods to your smoothies, whenever possible. For example:

-add a bit of dark chocolate or cocoa powder to your fruit vitamin-C rich smoothies (for example oranges, cocoa, coconut milk, and kiwi).

-add some hard-boiled eggs or meat/seafood leftovers to your vegetable vitamin-C rich smoothies (you can also use legumes, such as lentils or chickpeas, or nuts and seeds)

(for example: a smoothie made of red bell peppers, avocado, Himalayan salt, and some fresh tomato juice, can be made more filling by adding in some zinc-rich foods such as meat or seafood leftovers).

It's all about being creative and proactive. One simple meal can nourish your body with both Vitamin C and zinc while helping you save hours spent in your kitchen (and hundreds of dollars on expensive supplements that will not be effective anyways unless you take care of your diet first).

More zinc-rich recipes, including delicious salads and simple meal ideas such as...

Simple Spanish Tuna Salad

This delicious recipe is low in carbs, abundant in clean protein, and high in nutrients. It's also very rich in good fats to help you stay full and energized for hours!

Serves: 3-4

Ingredients:

•1 head of Romaine lettuce

•2 rip roma tomatoes, cut into wedges (however big you like)

•1 cucumber, peel and slice

•1 can asparagus (white)

•1 bell pepper, seed and slice into thin strips (lengthwise)

•1 avocado, peeled, pit and slice

•½ of a red onion, slice very thin

•1 carrot, grate

•2 hard-boiled eggs, peel and quarter (or trade for one can of albacore tuna in oil)

•red wine vinegar

•2-4 tablespoons extra virgin Spanish olive oil

•salt (to your liking)

•1 15 oz can artichoke hearts, drained

Instructions:

1.First, hard boil your two eggs. Then let them cool off in cold water and stick in freezer for a bit. When cool, peel and quarter.

2.Chop the whole romaine head in half and rinse and dry it.

3.Slice your tomatoes.

4.Slice cucumber after peeling.

5.Seed and the slice the peppers.

6.Grate carrot.

7.Open the cans of asparagus and artichokes and drain. Do the same if using tuna.

8.Tear up lettuce between two plates.

9.First lay on the tomato, then the cucumber, onion, pepper, and then carrots.

10.Break up the lettuce into small pieces for a salad. Make a bed of lettuce on a large platter. On top of the bed, place the tomatoes, cucumbers, onions, peppers and carrots. If using tuna spread it out around the lettuce.

11.Put the egg, asparagus, and artichoke on top.

12.Drizzle with oil and vinegar and salt to your liking.

Greek Breakfast Shrimp on Toast

I am not a big meat person, but I love seafood! Also, usually, I just have a quick smoothie for breakfast. However, I love this recipe for special and family occasions.

Serves 4

Ingredients:

• 1/3 cup olive oil

• 1 lb. shrimp (peel and de-vein)

• 4 minced garlic cloves

• 4 tomatoes (seed and chop)

• ½ chopped green onion

• ½ c. feta (crumble)

• ½ of a lemon squeezed

• 1 tbsp. dry oregano

• 1 tsp dry thyme

• 1 tsp dry basil

• 1 tsp dry marjoram

• 1 tsp each dry onion and garlic (minced)

• Mix and store in airtight container.

•Greek loaf sliced (gluten-free) into ½ in. slices

Instructions:

1.Place a large frying pan on the stove with 1 tablespoon oil and heat to medium high.

2.Add shrimp and garlic, sautéing for 4 min.

3.Remove from heat, place in a bowl, and chill.

4.Mix the tomatoes, 1 tablespoon olive oil, Greek seasoning, lemon juice, feta, and onion in another bowl and chill.

5.Take your bread slices and place them on a cookie sheet, brushing each one with olive oil. Place them in an oven set to 375 degrees Fahrenheit (or 190 Celsius) for 7-8 min.

6.When the bread is toasted, place some shrimp on each slice and top with tomato/cheese mixture.

7.Enjoy!

Egg-Lemon Tuna Soup

This recipe is original, tasty, nutritious and delicious. Tuna can make an amazing soup!

Serves 5-6

Ingredients:

- 3 carrots (chopped)

- 2 brown onions (chopped)

- 3-5 oz. cans tuna in oil (drained)

- 3 tablespoons fresh squeezed lemon juice

- ½ cup brown rice or quinoa

- 5 cups vegetable broth (stock)

- 1 cup water

- 1 tbsp extra virgin olive oil

- Himalayan salt to taste

- 3 organic eggs

Instructions:

1.Cook brown rice according to the package.

2.While that is cooking, put a medium sized pot on the stove and heat oil to medium-high. Add onion and sauté for 5 minutes.

3.Add the veggie broth and the water to the cooked onions and simmer.

4.When the rice is finished, add the it to the onion broth, along with the drained tuna. Allow to simmer for 7 minutes.

5.In a separate bowl, whisk the eggs well. Add the lemon juice while continuing to whisk. Keep whisking until well blended.

6.Next, ladle in one full scoop of broth, still whisking constantly with the other hand. Repeat one more time.

7.Take the soup pot off of the heat and whisk as you add the egg/broth into the pot.

8.Enjoy!

Arugula Tuna with Lemon Parsley Dressing

This salad offers an incredible mix of clean protein, good fats, and superfood greens. The alkaline keto way!

Serves: 2

Ingredients

For the Salad:

- 1 whole scallion, finely chopped

- 2 cups of fresh arugula, chopped

- 1 avocado, peeled, pitted and sliced

- Fresh chopped parsley for topping

- 2 cans of organic tuna in olive oil

For the dressing:

- 4 tablespoons of thick coconut milk

- 4 tablespoons of parsley, chopped

- 2 tablespoons organic lemon juice

- 2 pinches of Himalayan salt (you can always add more if you need to)

•A pinch of black pepper and chili (optional)

•1 big garlic clove, peeled

Instructions:

1. Combine all the salad ingredients in a big salad bowl and toss well.

2. Mix all the salad dressing ingredients using a small hand blender,

3. Pour the dressing over the salad and stir well.

5. Serve and enjoy!

Now, let's move on to the next of our Immune System Quartet Member – **Curcumin**.

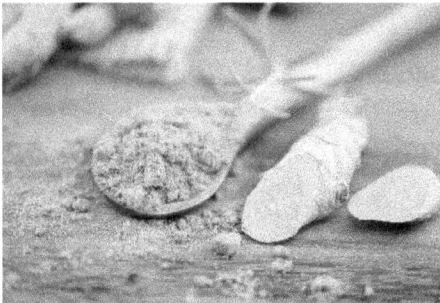

Curcumin is the key active ingredient in turmeric. It can be easily added to your diet through teas or smoothies.

I usually buy fresh turmeric root and add it to my herbal teas, soups or smoothies. Sometimes, I use a powdered curcumin supplement (with a little bit of black pepper) and also add it to my Vitamin C rich smoothies.

For example:

2 oranges + 1-inch grated turmeric (peeled)+ 1-inch ginger (peeled) + 1 tablespoon coconut oil + 1 cup coconut milk and a bit of cinnamon.

Blend and enjoy!

Pro tip – whenever peeling turmeric, be sure to use hand gloves to protect your fingers and nails from going orange!

Below, you will find some immune system boosting tea ideas that use turmeric!

These are very easy (you could even buy turmeric tea to enjoy at work!), and I am always looking forward to a nice, warm, healing and immune-system-boosting cup of tea!

Curcumin Herbal Tea Recipes to Boost Your Immune System

Fenugreek and Turmeric Dream

This recipe will help you feel lighter and more energized while protecting your immune system.

Serves: 1-2

Ingredients

•2 cups filtered water, boiling

•1 tbsp fenugreek seeds

•a few lime leaves, washed

•2 slices of lime

•a 1.5-inch piece of fresh turmeric root

•1 lemongrass stalk

Instructions

1.Bring the water to a boil using medium heat.

2.In the meantime, bash the fenugreek seeds a little, crush the lime leaves and cut the turmeric root.

3.Squash the lemongrass.

4.Add all the ingredients to boiling water. Reduce the heat to low.

5.Leave to simmer gently for 15-20 minutes so that the flavors get released.

6.Then, turn off the heat.

7.Strain all the ingredients and serve your tea in a nice teacup.

8.Garnish with some lime slices, enjoy!

Creamy Turmeric Latte

This one is delicious, creamy, healthy and guilt-free!

As an added bonus, this recipe will help you prevent sugar cravings…

Serves: 1-2

Ingredients

•1 cup cashew milk

•1 teaspoon cinnamon powder

•1 teaspoon turmeric powder

•1 teaspoon ginger powder

•1 teaspoon coconut oil

Instructions:

1.Place the milk in a pot and put to boil using medium heat.

2.Add cinnamon, turmeric, and ginger.

3.Stir well, cover and leave to simmer on low heat for about 10 minutes.

4.Pour into a cup and stir in a teaspoon of coconut oil.

5.Serve warm and enjoy!

Finally, let's have a look at Vitamin D3- the last member of our Healthy Immune System Boosting Quartet...

Vitamin D

Vitamin D is sometimes called the "sunshine vitamin" because it's produced in your skin in response to sunlight.

You can also get it through certain foods and, if needed, supplements to ensure adequate levels of the vitamin in your blood.

Getting a sufficient amount of vitamin D is important for normal growth and development of bones and teeth, as well as improved resistance against certain diseases.

The following foods are naturally rich in Vitamin D:

-Fatty fish, like tuna, mackerel, and salmon.

-Butter

-Beef liver

-Cheese.

-Egg yolks.

Now, let's have a look at some delicious recipes that are naturally rich in Vitamin D...

Spicy Ginger Salmon Salad

Ginger is well-known for its anti-inflammatory and healing properties. Cucumbers are highly refreshing and very nourishing. Salmon, avocado, nuts, and healthy oils will help you stay full for hours!

Serves: 2

Ingredients

For the Salad:

- 2 cucumbers, peeled and thinly sliced

- 1 tablespoon of grated ginger

- 1 cup arugula leaves

- 1 big avocado, peeled, pitted and sliced

- A handful of crushed almonds

- 2 slices of smoked salmon, cut into smaller pieces

For the Dressing:

- 1 tablespoon olive oil

- 1 tablespoon avocado oil

- 1 tablespoon fresh lime juice

•Black pepper to taste

•Himalayan salt to taste

To garnish:

•A few orange wedges

•A handful of cilantro leaves

Instructions:

1. Combine all the salad ingredients in a big salad bowl and toss well.

2. Mix all the salad dressing ingredients. You can use a small hand blender, or quickly combine and stir all the ingredients in a small bowl.

3. Pour the dressing over the salad and toss well.

4. Sprinkle over a handful of cilantro leaves and garnish with orange wedges.

5. Serve and enjoy!

Easy Creamy Warm Salmon Salad

Salmon is definitely one of my favorite Vitamin D-rich ingredients, especially to use for quick, nourishing salads like this one.

Servings: 1-2

Ingredients:

- Half cup raw cashews, crushed
- 4 slices of smoked salmon
- 2 tablespoons of coconut oil or butter
- 1 cup fresh spinach
- 2 tomatoes, sliced
- Himalaya salt and black pepper to taste
- A few thin slices of cheddar cheese

Instructions:

1. Place coconut oil in a frying pan.
2. Switch on the heat (medium heat).
3. Add the spinach and Himalaya salt and stir-fry until soft.
4. Now, add the salmon, cashews and tomato slices.
5. Stir fry until the salmon is warm.
6. Take off the heat and place in a salad bowl.
7. If needed, add more Himalaya salt to taste.
8. Top up with some cheddar cheese, serve and enjoy!

To sum up, our basic Immune System Quartet, If you are finding adding these supplements to your regimen is too expensive, all you need to focus on are:

-leafy greens,

-turmeric,

-and fatty fish!

Add some citric, Vitamin C-rich foods like lemons, limes, grapefruits, and oranges, and you are good to go.

Now, let's move on to the next step – your hydration and why it's so important. I will also share with you how I now manage to save up around 1000 dollars a year by doing this step!

Staying healthy is one thing. But doing it and saving money at the same time is even better!

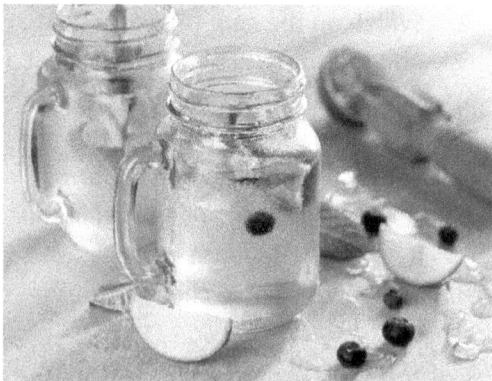

Proper Hydration (and how it can help you save money and even lose weight!)

You can't have a properly-functioning, strong immune system if you are dehydrated. This is super important, and the good news, it doesn't have to be expensive.

It can help you save money in the long run.

But...I know what you're thinking...how much water is enough...and what 'type' of water/filter.?

First question: how much is enough? Well, to keep this simple – for most people, drinking between 2.5 – 4 liters (85fl oz – 135fl oz) a day is a good recommendation. Aim for around 3 liters / 100 fl oz per day as a guide and adjust it depending on your lifestyle, or the climate you live in (needless to say- you feel like drinking more water if it's hot, or if you are exercising).

Winter can be a bit tricky. Why? Because your body will be naturally craving something warm and forcing yourself to drink lots of water can be a bit of a challenge. The best way to fix it, is to:

-focus on warm, herbal infusions

-Spice up your water with some lemon or lime juice and add in a bit of a warm herbal infusion (or warm, but not boiling) water – more on that later, in the healing tea section.

For now, let's focus on the basics. Let's set a goal of drinking around 3 liters / 100 fl oz per day as a guide.

Yes, this may seem like a lot, to begin with, but don't worry, it's not so hard if you start tweaking your lifestyle, step-by-step.

If you are drinking nothing but coffee and tea (caffeinated tea like black tea or green tea) at the moment, don't go from zero to 100fl oz in one day (unless you want to). Start by having 40 a day, then after a few days up to 80, then up to 100, and so on.

If you are not a big fan of plain water, feel free to infuse it with some delicious (and Vitamin C rich) fruits. I love infusing my water with fruits.

Another great way to stay hydrated is to add herbal infusions. We are talking caffeine-free teas and infusions such as:

-fennel tea (also great to strengthen your immune system)

-mint (great for your digestion and overall refreshment)

-chamomile

-turmeric or ginger tea

Please note- while regular tea (such as black tea) and coffee is OK in moderation, they do not count as water or hydrating liquids as they do the opposite.

However, herbal teas, make it very easy to stay hydrated. I usually drink 3-4 big cups of herbal tea a day (all kinds of teas, for variety), which equals to 1 liter of water a day.

That's already one-third of our goal. I also sip on lemon water in between my meals and, as I have already mentioned, I am also a big lover of smoothies and nut milk (they are also very hydrating).

However, the goal number one here is your Water Habit.

If you're dehydrated all the time now, you will need to pee a lot, the first time when you increase your intake of water. But this will subside after a week, after your body gets used to it, maybe less. You might also get MORE thirsty the more you drink – go with the flow and drink more!

Now, our next question is - what type of water do I need to drink? It all comes down to understating a few simple guidelines:

-Avoid bottled water – all kinds of bottled water, even if it says "alkalized" or "magnesium/ calcium added". It's not a miracle nor a cure. It is very expensive and over-hyped. It's terrible for the environment and is likely poorly filtered. Bottled water companies have less strict guidelines than tap water companies. At the same time – plastic is toxic and full of chemicals – so be sure to avoid it.

Also, keep in mind that many bottles are not BPA-free.

And even if they are – your water is still stored in plastic for months before you drink it, which is very unhealthy.

There are many legit alkaline water ionizers that get plenty of good reviews, but they are pretty expensive. Also, if you rent a place, you might not be able to change the entire installation.

If you already have one- great, keep using it!

So, the most effective solution I found is a simple filtration system - a regular counter-top filter jug will suffice. We use the one Britta (you can get it on Amazon very inexpensively), and it helps us save a lot of money on bottled water and sodas.

This is the most affordable and effective solution! I filter my water and add in a bit of lemon or lime juice. It's naturally low in sugar and high in Vitamin C. And, believe it or not, ever since I started using this simple system, I have been losing weight. Why?

-I stopped drinking sugar and calorie-rich sodas and other fizzy drinks or sugar-high processed fruit juices (because of that, my sugar cravings massively reduced, pretty much naturally!).

-I regained my energy naturally, and found the motivation to work out and go out for long walks

-My body began releasing toxins (lemon water is very detoxifying) and letting go of fat, as a result.

Don't take my word for it! Try it yourself!

Now that you know what kind of water to use, let's have a look at some original, immune-system-boosting recipes.

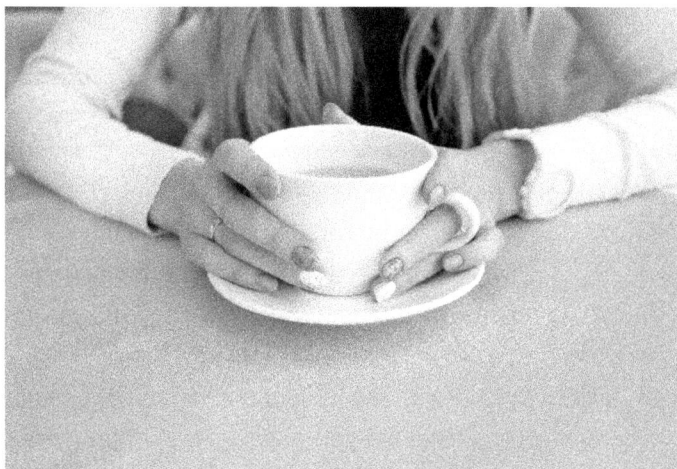

Ginger and Turmeric Tea

This tea is great for getting rid of coughs and colds. It's spicy, comforting, and absolutely delicious.

Serves: 1
Ingredients:
- 1-inch ginger, peeled
- 1-inch turmeric, peeled
- 1 cup water, boiling
- 1 Indian spice blend tea bag
- 1 teaspoon honey

Instructions:
1. Place all the tea ingredients (except honey) in a teapot and pour over some boiling water.
2. Keep covered for 15 minutes.
3. Strain and serve warm (but not boiling) in a tea cup with 1 teaspoon of honey.

Note: If you are unable to find the Indian spice tea bags then you can prepare your own. To prepare the tea bag mix together tea leaves along with a couple of cloves, 1 black cardamom pod, 1 teaspoon black pepper corns, ½ inch cinnamon stick and a few green cardamom pods.

Easy Chili Tea

This tea will help in cleansing your digestive tract while warming you up and giving you a strong energy boost that will last for hours.

Serves: 2
Ingredients:

- 2 cups water, boiling
- 2 fennel tea bags
- 2 red chili flakes
- A handful of fresh mint leaves
- 2 tablespoons honey

Instructions:

1. Place all the tea ingredients (except honey) in a teapot and pour over 2 cups of boiling water.
2. Keep covered for 15 minutes.
3. Strain and serve warm (but not boiling) in a teacup with 1 teaspoon of honey.

Cumin and Caraway Tea

Aside from helping you boost your immune system, this tea is great for those women looking to obtain relief from period cramps.

Serves: 1-2
Ingredients:
- 2 cups water, boiling
- 1 black tea bag (optional, if you need an energy boost but you can skip it if you want to keep it 100% caffeine-free)
- 1 inch ginger, peeled
- 1 tablespoon cumin seeds
- 1 tablespoon caraway seeds
- 1 tablespoon coriander seeds
- 1 tablespoon fennel seeds
- 1 tablespoon honey, if needed

Instructions:
1. Place all the tea ingredients (except honey) in a tea pot and pour over 2 cups of boiling water.
2. Keep covered for 15 minutes.
3. Strain and serve warm (but not boiling) in a tea cup with 1 teaspoon of honey.

Spicy Chai Tea

This tea is super tasty and creamy. It can be consumed on a regular basis, and it's great to prevent colds too.

Serves: 1-2

Ingredients:

- 1 cup almond or coconut milk
- 1 Indian chai tea bag
- 2-inch turmeric, peeled
- 2 tablespoons honey

Instructions:

1. Boil almond milk using a saucepan
2. When boiling, add the teabag and turmeric.
3. Simmer on low heat for 5 minutes.
4. Turn off the heat and keep covered for 15 minutes.
5. Pour into a teacup and sweeten with honey if needed

In the absence of chai tea, make use of tea leaves mixed with cinnamon, cloves, and cardamon. Make it sweet and healthy by adding almond milk.

Ashwagandha Tea

This is a great Ayurvedic tea to help you stay hydrated while boosting your immune system.

Serves: 1-2
Ingredients:
- 1 tablespoon dried ashwagandha
- 2 cups water, boiling
- 1 fennel tea bag
- 1 green tea bag
- 1 tablespoon honey (optional)

Instructions:
1. Place all the tea ingredients (except honey) in a teapot and pour over some boiling water.
2. Keep covered for 15 minutes.
3. Strain and serve warm (but not boiling) in a tea cup with 1 teaspoon of honey (if needed)

Now, let's move on to the next step...proper sleep

Sleep – Quality Over Quantity?

Even though sleep is free, most people ignore it. However, we need to remember that sleep is one of the most important factors for strengthening your immune system. Yes, I know, sleep can be hard—stress, family obligations, little kids, or not enough time. I understand!

Let's move back to our first health pillar – empowerment. What was our empowerment all about?

Well, it was all about focusing on solutions instead of excuses. And it's all about doing the best we can.

Let's have a look at some facts:

A sleep-deprived immune system does not function well. In one study conducted in 2015, 164 men and women were assessed for their duration of sleep and susceptibility to the cold virus. Yep, strangely these 164 participants were happy to be given the cold!

The results made it clear, that not everyone got sick, but those who had less than 6-hour sleep a night were over 400% more likely to. The risk was even higher when a person slept less than five hours a night.

So, promise yourself to do the best you can by optimizing your sleep by:

-avoid caffeine after lunch (if you are very nervous, I would recommend you cut down on coffee entirely or reduce it to one small cup very early in the morning- then drink lemon water and herbal tea only).

-avoid screen within 60-120 minutes of sleep.

I used to struggle with sleep, and when a friend told me about meditation, I quickly rejected it as some "woo-woo". But, eventually, I gave it a try, and after doing some research, I have learned that regular meditation can help your body rejuvenate faster. Also, when you meditate, your body is already at a deep, relaxed state, and some meditation teachers and researchers even say that the more you meditate, the less sleep you need.

I wouldn't go so far in claims (unless you have tested it, it works for you, and you're happy with it). You still need your sleep. But, from my experience, regular meditation, especially evening meditation, helps me relax and sleep better.

So, instead of scrolling my Facebook and Instagram, feed, I listen to some relaxing music, switch off my phone and meditate until I get so sleepy (and relaxed) that falling asleep is no longer a problem.

If you are looking for inexpensive supplements to help you sleep better, I would recommend:

-Ashwagandha powder (I also have a book on Ashwagandha herb, if you want to check it out).

-lavender and Melissa tea

-inhaling lavender essential oil (through a diffuser- it also helps to purify the air)

-an Epsom salt bath (I also have a book on it, if you want to give it a go), with some coconut oil and a few drops of lavender oil

-Magnesium supplement (if prescribed by your doctor) or Magnesium-rich foods (avocados, Himalayan salt, and healthy smoothies with greens will help you boost your Magnesium intake naturally and almost effortlessly).

Lavender essential oils and Epsom salt can be purchased very inexpensively on Amazon. You can also download many free meditations online, including meditations with music, or guided meditations. There are also many meditations recorded by hypnosis experts, aimed at eliminating insomnia, stress and anxiety.

Now, let's have a look at a few more recipes to help you sleep better!

Sleep Well Tea

This recipe will help you unwind after a busy day, sleep like a baby, and wake up feeling energized.

Serves: 2

Ingredients

- 1 cup of water, boiling
- 1 lemongrass stalk
- 2 tablespoons chamomile tea
- A few tablespoons of coconut milk
- 1 tablespoon of coconut oil
- A dash of cinnamon powder to garnish

Instructions:

1. Place all the tea ingredients (except coconut milk and oil) in a tea pot and pour over some boiling water.
2. Keep covered for 15 minutes.
3. Strain.
4. Pour into a tea cup and add in the coconut milk and oil.
5. Stir well.
6. Sprinkle over some cinnamon powder, enjoy!

Easy Mediterranean Tea Template

Rosemary and fennel are both miraculous herbs and will help you boost your immune system and fight off colds and flu.

Fennel is also great for weight loss as well as stimulating your lymphatic system.

Serves:2

Ingredients:

- 2 cups boiling water
- 1 tablespoon rosemary herb
- 1 tablespoon fennel seeds
- 1 teaspoon Melissa tea (optional)

Instructions:

1. Place all the tea ingredients (except honey) in a tea pot and pour over some boiling water.
2. Keep covered for 15 minutes.
3. Strain and serve warm (but not boiling) in a tea cup with 1 teaspoon of honey (if needed)

More Immune-Boosting Foods to Focus On

Greens – Eat Them, Blend Them, Juice Them...Whatever Works for You!

Greens are the most nutrient-dense foods you can get. The good news? They are very inexpensive!

So, if you want to boost your immune system, add more greens into your diet. We are talking:

-spinach

-lettuce

-kale

-arugula

If you are not a salad person- focus on green smoothies.

And, if you are not a smoothie person, focus on snacking on some greens (such as kale) with hummus, or add them to your salads.

The recipes below (smoothies and salads) will give you some ideas so that you can start taking action as soon as possible.

Vitamin C Energy and Mood Boosting Smoothie

Having a bad day? Do you need to boost your mood? Try this smoothie. It offers a healthy mix of vitamin C, energy stimulating greens, and mood-boosting cocoa.

Servings: 1-2
Ingredients
Liquid:
- 1 cup coconut milk or gluten-free rice milk (unsweetened)
- Half cup water, filtered, preferably alkaline water
- 1 teaspoon coconut oil

Dry:
- 1-inch ginger, peeled
- 1-inch turmeric, peeled
- Half cup arugula leaves
- 1 orange, peeled

Other:
- Stevia to sweeten (optional)
- Half teaspoon cinnamon
- 1 tablespoon cocoa powder
- 1 tablespoon chia seeds
- A few drops of liquid chlorophyll (optional)

Instructions:
1. Blend and enjoy.
2. Add some stevia to sweeten if needed.
3. This drink is great first thing in the morning. But you can also sip on it during the day to enjoy more energy or whenever you are having a bad day!

Green Almond Protein Hormone Balancer

This delicious smoothie uses maca powder, which is a hormone re-balancer for women.

Servings: 1-2
Ingredients
Liquid:

- 1 cup coconut or almond milk (unsweetened)
- 1 tablespoon coconut oil
- Half cup coconut water

Dry:

- Half cup kale leaves
- 1 banana, peeled
- Half green apple

Other:

- A bit of stevia to sweeten
- Half teaspoon fresh maca powder
- 1 tablespoon hemp seed protein powder (personally, I like chocolate-flavored protein powder)

+ a few lime slices and ice cubes to serve if needed

Instructions:

1. Place all the ingredients in a blender.
2. Process until smooth.
3. Serve and enjoy!
4. This smoothie also tastes delicious when chilled or half-frozen.

Simple Detox Spicy Smoothie

If you are looking for a quick detox recipe-this smoothie recipe will help you sweat out all the toxins and supercharge your nutrition!

Servings: 2-3
Ingredients
Liquid:
- 1 cup organic tomato juice
- Half cup unsweetened almond milk

Dry:
- 2 big cucumbers, peeled and roughly sliced
- 6 radishes, sliced
- 2 tablespoons chive, chopped
- 1 garlic clove, peeled
- Half cup arugula leaves, washed
- 1 teaspoon hemp protein powder

Other:
- Pinch of Himalayan salt
- Pinch of black pepper
- Pinch of chili powder

Instructions:
1. Place all the ingredients through a blender.
2. Blend, serve, and enjoy!

You can also serve this smoothie as a quick, raw soup and add in some quality protein of your choice (hard-boiled eggs or meat leftovers).

Turmeric & Ginger – Inexpensive and Super Effective!

The gingerols in ginger and curcumin in turmeric are probably two of the most anti-inflammatory compounds ever invented. And, it's all-natural! They also contain powerful antioxidants too, and support the body's stress response for a healthier lifestyle.

Start adding some ginger or turmeric to your tea today! You can also juice ginger (if you have a juicer) and start adding ginger juice to your water, smoothies, and other healthy beverages.

Ginger and turmeric also taste great in soups and all kinds of healthy, vegetable stir-fries.

Your Healing Ginger Soup

This recipe is simple, creamy, and so incredibly aromatic!

Servings: 2

Ingredients:

• 2-inch ginger, peeled and minced

• 2 big garlic cloves, minced

• 1 tablespoon coconut oil

•2 tablespoons nut butter of choice (personally, I love some fresh, home-made cashew butter)

•1 cup coconut milk

•Half cup water, filtered, preferably alkaline

•3 orange wedges

•3 large chopped carrots

Instructions:

1.Start off by frying the ginger and garlic in coconut oil, using a medium-sized pan.

2.While enjoying the aroma (nothing smells better than stir-fried ginger), proceed to blend the carrots, orange wedges, coconut milk, nut butter, and water.

3.Blend until creamy.

4.Now, add the mixture to the frying ginger and garlic, reduce to low heat, and stir for a few minutes.

5.Serve lightly warm and enjoy!

Garlic – The Most Powerful Natural Antibiotic

Garlic is a powerful immune-booster, mostly because of the compound allicin. Garlic has been shown to lower LDL cholesterol; it's a powerful antibiotic and anti-viral.

However, the allicin is hugely present in RAW garlic, and it disappears quickly once it's exposed to air or cooked.

So, if you want to use garlic to boost your immune system, I highly recommend focusing on raw garlic. You can easily do it by:

-adding some garlic to your salads, or blending it into your salad dressings

-adding it to your veggie creams or hummus (as well as pesto and other dips)

Garlic also tastes great in vegetable smoothies!

Anti-Flu Green Smoothie

This recipe uses healing, mineral-rich veggies like cauliflower, and, at the same time, adds in some garlic to help you strengthen your immune system.

Servings: 1-2
Ingredients
Liquid:

- 2 cups almond milk
- 1 tablespoon olive oil

Dry:

- half cup cauliflower, slightly cooked or steamed, cut into smaller pieces
- 2 garlic cloves, peeled and minced
- 1 cup arugula leaves
- One small chili flake (optional)

Other:

- Himalaya salt
- Half teaspoon curry powder
- Half teaspoon turmeric powder with a pinch of black pepper
- 1 teaspoon chlorella

Instructions:

1. Place all the ingredients in a blender.
2. Blend until smooth, serve and enjoy!

Avocado -Another Effective Immune-System Boosting Superfood

I highly recommend you increase your intake of healthy fats (omega 3 and saturated fat from coconut oil or avocado) to support your overall health and immunity.

Avocado contains the highest concentration of L-glutathione, known as the "master antioxidant". Glutathione is essential because it enables all other antioxidants to function, protect cells against free radical damage, and detoxifies the body of pollutants and other toxins.

It's also very rich in Magnesium to help your body stay in balance.

The best way to make sure you consume enough of avocados is to:

-enjoy them raw (with some Himalayan salt, pepper, and other spices of your choice)

-Use it in smoothies, soups, salads, wraps – get it in however you can.

-Add them to your smoothies! You can make delicious and naturally creamy, super healthy smoothies such as:

-1 avocado + 1 cup of nut milk + a bit of cinnamon powder + a few banana slices (so yummy and healthy!).

Below are some delicious avocado-salad ideas:

Nourishing Herbal Avocado Salad

The herbs used in this salad make avocado taste amazing, and they also add to the mineral and nutrient content of this salad.

Serves: 2

Ingredients:

•2 avocados, peeled, halved and pitted

•¼ cup of mixed Mediterranean herbs (for example thyme, rosemary, basil, oregano, parsley)

•¼ cup of dried cherry tomatoes, quartered

•¼ cup of cooked chickpeas or black beans

•Optional: 1 sheet of nori, cut into smaller pieces

•1 tablespoon of extra virgin avocado oil

•Juice of half lemon

•Pinch of black pepper and Himalaya salt to taste, if needed

Instructions:

1.Place the avocado halves in a serving bowl.

2.Add the rest of the ingredients.

3.Drizzle with some avocado oil and lemon juice.

4.If needed, season with Himalaya salt and black pepper.

5.Enjoy!

Avocado Strawberries Salad

This recipe shows the versatility of the avocado. It also shows how well it can blend with both sweet ingredients like strawberries with the mustardy flavor of the rocket (arugula).

It's also a fantastic way to sneak in more greens into your diet.

Serves: 1-2

Ingredients:

• 1 big ripe avocado, pitted and sliced

• 1 cup of fresh strawberries, quartered

• Half cup of raw pecan nuts, roughly chopped

•Half cup of fresh rocket (arugula) leaves, finely chopped

•2 tablespoons of thick coconut milk

•1 tablespoon of raw seed mix

•1 tablespoon of coconut shavings

Instructions:

1.In a bowl, combine the strawberries, avocado, pecan nuts, fresh rocket (arugula), raw seed mix and the coconut milk.

2.Toss together.

3.Sprinkle over the coconut shavings and serve.

4.Enjoy!

Grilled Chicken Salad with Grapefruit and Avocado

This yummy dish is served with delicious low-sugar, Vitamin C fruits. It's perfect as a quick, comforting dinner recipe.

Serves:2-3

Ingredients

For the Salad:

• 4 skinless chicken breast halves (remove the bones)

• 8 cups of mixed salad greens

• 1 cup of grapefruit chunks

• 3/4th cup of avocado, peeled and diced

• 3/4th teaspoon of grated fresh ginger

For the Dressing:

• 2 tablespoons of low carb mango chutney

• 2 tablespoons of olive oil

• 2 tablespoons of fresh lime juice

•1 tablespoon of coconut aminos

•Cooking spray

Instructions:

1.Preheat a grill and grease it with some cooking spray.

2.Take a bowl and combine the coconut aminos, chutney, lime juice, olive oil, and ginger in it. Keep aside.

3.Lay the chicken breast halves on a flat surface and brush those with 2 tablespoons of the chutney mixture.

4.Grill the chicken for 4 minutes on each side while coating lightly with the chutney mixture again on flipping. Remove from grill once done.

5.Cut the chicken into diagonal pieces. Lay the avocado slices, grapefruit, and salad greens on the plate and place the chicken pieces on top to serve. Enjoy!

Again, you don't have to do all of this perfectly from day one. I know it's a lot of info and recipes! I don't want you to feel overwhelmed (feeling overwhelmed hardly ever leads to taking action!). So, just relax and add some of these in as you can and commit to doing a little more each day. Also, the more you focus on adding, the easier it will be for you to let go or reduce the foods that are not serving you and your immune system...

The Most Immune-Suppressing Foods to Avoid

Yes, since it is a wellness book aimed at healthy eating,

I am sure you were expecting me to tell you which foods you need to start letting go of. Well, this booklet is structured the way it is for a reason. Why?

Personally, I find it a lot easier to add some healthy foods before reducing the unhealthy ones.

Of course, the best thing to do, would be to do the two at the same time – focus both on reducing the bad foods and adding the good ones.

However, what most people do wrong is that they start cutting out all the unhealthy foods and drinks using will power alone. The result? Your body is confused. You are not putting anything nourishing in it. All you are focusing on is elimination, "cutting out this and that", and "being on a diet". So, what happens? Well, your body begins craving bad foods again, because it feels hungry and deprived.

It's so much easier to let go or reduce the unhealthy foods, if your main focus is nourishing your body with super healthy, nutrient-rich superfoods (like the foods and recipes we have covered in this book!).

So now, let's focus on foods that are weakening your immune system...

Food to Avoid #1: SUGAR

Sugar is the most pro-inflammatory, immune-suppressing, hormone-unbalancing substance ever created. In fact, it's more addictive than cocaine!

If you want to stay healthy and take care of your immune system, quit the sugar or reduce it as much as possible.

The problem? If you eat processed and packaged foods – the sugar is almost everywhere. Then, milk and dairy products also contain sugar. So do fruit juices (even home-made)!

Hence, my earlier tip – fruit is good for you as it's rich in Vitamin C your immune system needs every day.

However, try to focus on low-sugar fruit more than high-sugar-fruit. If you choose high sugar fruit, then eat it as a snack, in between your meals (one thing for sure, it's much better for you than candy or chocolate bars!).

You can also add a bit of high sugar fruit to your smoothies, especially your green smoothies to make them taste nicer.

However (and this is a very big however), if you like fresh juices, focus on vegetable juices or juices made of low sugar fruit. For example, lemon, lime, or grapefruit juice is much better for you than pure orange juice. Why? Well, oranges are higher in sugar than limes and lemons. And so, if you juice them, you take their fiber away, which makes it easier for your body to absorb all the contents from the juice, including – the sugar!

Also, drinking fruit juice made from high sugar fruit will make you crave even more sugar (and can also make you feel bloated).

And yes, I love oranges! But I don't juice them. I put them in my smoothies instead, as the fiber protects our body from overdoing the sugar. Fiber fills you up, and so, there is a limit to how many smoothies you can drink, or how many fruits you can eat.

With juices – they taste nice and sweet. There is no fiber, and so it's easy to drink even 2 big cups of orange juice in one sitting (or more!). That equals to about 45 grams of sugar. The same as in 10-12 teaspoons of sugar, how crazy is that!

Oh, yes, I can hear some angry voices from some of you, my fastidious readers!

But, sugar from orange juice is healthy and natural!

Well, it's STILL sugar. Your body doesn't care. It treats all forms and sources of sugar equally.

At the same time, one orange is only 9-10 grams sugar and can be a great addition to your smoothies, or a great, natural, vitamin C snack.

However, it takes many oranges to make 2 cups of orange juice (and ingest about 42-45 grams of sugar as a result).

These are what I like to call the Invisible Culprits. We learn about the dangers of sugar, and we stop putting sugar in our coffee, we quit sugary snacks and cut down on chocolate...

But then, we still consume sugar with many packed foods, yoghurts, and juice made of high sugar fruits. Most sauces and condiments also contain insane amounts of sugar. Our nation is running on sugar; they put sugar almost everywhere. The only solution is to start transitioning to a clean and whole-food lifestyle.

I have written many cookbooks and healthy recipe guides, including Paleo Salads, and Alkaline Keto Book series. You can find them on Amazon as well as on our website:

www.YourWellnessBooks.com/books

Food to Avoid #2: GLUTEN

Once again, living a healthy lifestyle and focusing on natural, clean, and whole-some foods (that all healthy diets, including: Paleo, Keto, Plant-based etc) preach, will help you reduce gluten and swap it with much healthier alternatives.

Gluten-containing grains (lust like their good buddy, Mr.Sugar) are the most pro-inflammatory, acid-forming, immune-suppressing substance on Earth.!

Gluten also has the added evil of directly leading to autoimmune. The breakdown of gluten's two proteins, gliadin and glutenin in the small intestine leads to a third protein being produced, zonulin.

That causes tears to appear in the small intestine (aka leaky gut) – which leads to food passing back into the bloodstream, and there you have it – autoimmune).

The gluten-containing grains to avoid include:

-Wheat

-Barley

-Rye

-Spelt

-Kamut

-Farro

-Bulgur

Please read the labels, as many foods, even though labeled as healthy and organic, do contain gluten!

Instead, use these naturally gluten-free alternatives:

-Oats (certified gluten-free)

-Chia

-Quinoa

-Coconut, almond, tiger nut (for flour etc)

-Sprouted grains – sprouted wheat etc. contains no gluten

Gluten-free cereals, pastas, bread are easy to get these days.

You can also use zucchini noodles instead of spaghetti…quinoa instead of barley etc.

Personally, I just focus on Paleo, Keto, and Alkaline foods as much as possible, as these are all naturally gluten-free!

This is why all my healthy eating books are inspired by these diets.

We very often crave gluten and sugar because we want a treat. Something sweet and delicious. Well, I have some good news for you! You can make these naturally gluten-free (and sugar-free) recipes instead!

As an added bonus, their nutrient-rich content will help you strengthen your body and fortify your immune system.

Totally Guilt Free, Sugar-Free, Gluten-Free Snacks

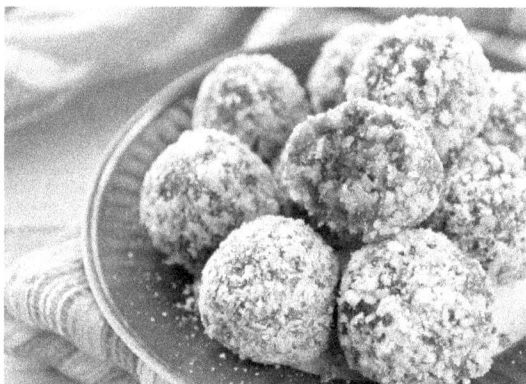

Ridiculously Easy Sweet Balls

Ingredients:

- 1 cup raw cashews (unsalted, unsweetened), soaked for at least 4 hours
- 1 cup raw almonds (unsalted, unsweetened), soaked for at least 4 hours
- 4 tablespoons coconut oil
- 4 tablespoons coconut milk
- 1 tablespoon cinnamon powder

Instructions:

1. Place all the ingredients in a high-speed blender or a food processor.
2. Using your hands, form the "dough" into small balls.
3. Place the balls on a big plate and put in a fridge for a few hours.
4. Serve and enjoy!

Creamy Sweet Alkaline Keto Porridge

This recipe is perfect if you are craving something sweet and creamy. It's super easy to make.

Servings: 2

Ingredients:

- 1 cup raw cashews
- 1 cup of coconut milk
- 2 tablespoons coconut oil
- 1 tablespoon cinnamon powder
- 1 tablespoon chia seeds
- Optional: 1 teaspoon maca powder
- A few blueberries to garnish

Instructions:

1. Combine all the ingredients in a bowl.
2. Mix well, serve and enjoy!

Delicious Chia Pudding Recipe

I came up with this recipe by accident. Just using the ingredients, I had available. To my surprise, the result was really delicious (and super healthy). This guilt-free treat is loaded with fiber, Iron, calcium, and omega-3 fatty acids. After all, chia seeds are one of the most nutritious foods on the planet and are just perfect for treats, smoothies and all kinds of creamy recipes.

Servings: 2

Ingredients:

- 1 cup unsweetened full-fat coconut milk
- Half teaspoon liquid stevia to sweeten (it's optional though, you can do very well without it)
- Half teaspoon vanilla extract
- Half teaspoon cinnamon powder
- Half cup fresh blackberries, preferably organic
- 4 tablespoons chia seeds
- Optional: half teaspoon maca powder
- Optional: half teaspoon ginger powder

Instructions:

1. Process all the ingredients using a blender or a food processor.
2. If needed, process a few times to make sure you obtain a smooth mixture.
3. Now, divide the mixture between two small cups with lids, and refrigerate overnight (or, for at least a few hours).
4. Serve and enjoy, it's really delicious!

BONUS: The Shots of Health – No Juicer Needed – Juice & Drink Recipes

Simple Chlorophyll Juice

This juice is great for boosting your energy and stimulating weight loss. Liquid chlorophyll is a fantastic way of enriching your juice with more nutrients, and it's perfect if you are too busy to juice the heaps of greens. To make this recipe, you don't even need an Omega Juicer, you could easily do with a simple lemon squeezer.

If you are looking for liquid chlorophyll, or green powder recommendation, please check our website:

www.YourWellnessBooks.com/resources

Servings: 2

Ingredients:

- 2 big grapefruits
- 1 cup thick coconut milk, full fat, unsweetened
- 1 tablespoon avocado oil
- Half teaspoon cinnamon powder

- A few drops of liquid chlorophyll (optional)
- Stevia to sweeten- optional

Instructions:

1. Juice the grapefruits (a lemon squeezer tool like the one on the picture below, will do for this recipe).
2. Combine the juice with avocado oil, coconut milk, cinnamon powder, and liquid chlorophyll.
3. Stir well, serve in a glass and enjoy!

Green Tea Bullet Proof Vitamin C Juice

This recipe uses green tea to help you boost your energy levels and burn fat. Ginger adds to anti-inflammatory properties. Then, there is grapefruit, super-rich in Vitamin C, and alkaline minerals.

That mix combines really well with coconut oil. So tasty and good for you! Once again, for this recipe, you don't even need a fancy juicer. A simple lemon squeezer will do.

Servings: 2

Ingredients:

- 1 big grapefruit
- 1-inch ginger, peeled
- 1 cup green tea, cooled down (use 1 teabag per cup)
- 2 tablespoons coconut oil
- Stevia to sweeten if needed

Instructions:

1.Make the green tea, add in ginger, and leave covered to boil.

2.In the meantime, juice grapefruit using a lemon squeezer or a juicer.

3.In a small hand blender, combine the grapefruit juice and coconut oil. Process until smooth.

4.Once the green tea cools down, pour the juice into a big glass or a jar, and combine with the tea. Serve as it is or chilled. Enjoy!

Grapefruit juice benefits:

-helps in weight loss (it's low in calories and high in nutrients)

-very low in carbs and sugars

-stimulates the lymphatic system, helping you feel lighter and more energized

-boost the immune system

Your Healthy Immune System-Boosting Drink Templates (no juicer needed)

This template will help you come up with your own recipes!

You need:

-Lemons, limes, or grapefruits squeezed (use a simple lemon squeezer) – you can also use more than 1.

-filtered water, or herbal infusion, or coconut milk (or any other nut milk) – you can also use more than 1.

-optional – liquid chlorophyll, powdered greens, or maca powder (you can find some of our recommendations on our website:

www.YourWellnessBooks.com/resources)

Remember. Your body is smart. It wants to stay healthy and keep you happy. You just need to nourish it from the inside out!

We are in this together,

Thank you for reading to the end,

Elena

We Need Your Help

One more thing, before you go, could you please do us a quick favor?

It would be great if you could leave us a short review on Amazon.

Don't worry, it doesn't have to be long. One sentence is enough.

Let others know your favorite recipes and who you think this book can help.

Thank You for your support!

(if you have any questions about this book, you can also email us at: info@yourwellnessbooks.com)

Join Our VIP Readers' Newsletter to Boost Your Wellbeing

Would you like to be notified about our new health and wellness books? How about receiving them at deeply discounted prices? What about awesome giveaways, latest health tips, and motivation? If that is something you are interested in, please visit the link below to join our newsletter:

www.yourwellnessbooks.com/email-newsletter

As a bonus, you will receive a free complimentary eBook *Alkaline Paleo Superfoods*

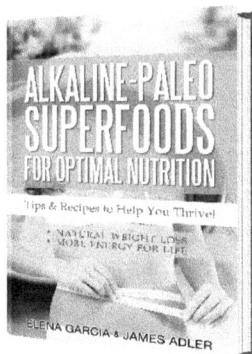

Sign up link:

www.yourwellnessbooks.com/email-newsletter

More Books & Resources in the Healthy Lifestyle Series
Available at:

www.yourwellnessbooks.com

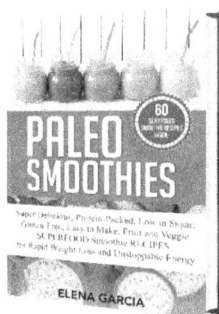

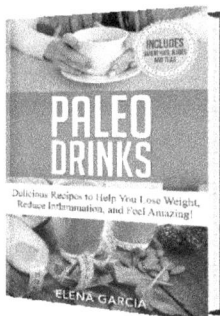

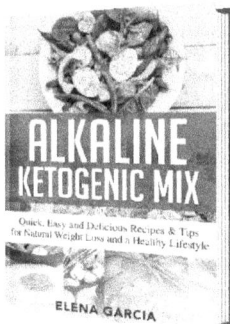

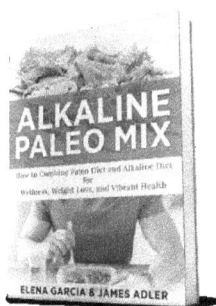

www.ingramcontent.com/pod-product-compliance
Lightning Source LLC
Chambersburg PA
CBHW051030030426
42336CB00015B/2811